ACUPUNCTURE POINT FOR BEGINNERS

Unlocking Wellness, A Beginner's Guide To Explore, Discover The Key Techniques, Focus Areas, And Major Targets For Health And Balance

LAMBERT FETTERMAN

All rights reserved. Except for brief quotations embodied in critical reviews and certain other noncommercial uses permitted by copyright law, no part of this book may be reproduced, distributed, or transmitted in any form or by any means, including photocopying, recording, or other electronic or mechanical methods, without the prior written permission of the author.

DISCLAIMER

The content in this book is offered only for general informative purposes. While every effort has been taken to guarantee the content's accuracy and completeness, the author and publisher accept no responsibility for any mistakes or omissions, or for the results of using the information given herein. The methods, recommendations, and directions in this book are not guaranteed to be appropriate for every person, and readers should exercise caution and seek professional counsel if required before undertaking any of the projects or techniques detailed in this book.

Table of Contents

INTRODUCTION

Understanding The Basics Of Acupuncture

Acupuncture is an ancient Chinese medicinal procedure in which small needles are inserted into precise places on the body to relieve pain and enhance general well-being.

Acupuncture's primary theory focuses on the flow of energy, known as Qi (pronounced "chee"), along routes in the body known as meridians. Practitioners attempt to restore health by stimulating particular sites along these meridians.

History And Origins Of Acupuncture

For thousands of years, acupuncture has been employed in Chinese medicine. Its roots are entrenched in history and philosophy, and it has evolved over centuries. Early practitioners discovered that stimulating certain areas of the body might relieve pain and heal a variety of diseases. The ideas and practices of acupuncture were chronicled in ancient books such as the Yellow Emperor's Classic of Internal Medicine (Huangdi Neijing).

How Acupuncture Works

Acupuncture's basic premise focuses on the balance of Yin and Yang, opposing energies that need equilibrium for maximum health.

The body maintains in balance when Qi circulates freely throughout the meridians, but interruptions in this flow may cause sickness or pain. Acupuncture attempts to restore this balance by focusing on particular points, stimulating the body's natural healing processes, and promoting general well-being.

CHAPTER 1

The Human Body And Energy Pathways

Exploring Meridians

Meridians are Qi circulation channels. Twelve principal meridians run along the body's surface, each connected with a unique organ system. Understanding these meridians is important because acupuncturists use these channels to treat health problems.

Organ Systems And Their Corresponding Meridians

Each principal meridian corresponds to a different organ system in the body. The Lung meridian, for example, is associated with the respiratory system, the Liver meridian with cleansing and digestion, and so on. Understanding these relationships helps in the diagnosis and treatment of diseases.

Understanding Qi: Vital Energy Flow

The vital energy that travels through the meridians is known as qi. It is thought that health is maintained when Qi flows easily and harmoniously. Disruptions or obstructions in this flow might result in sickness or pain. Acupuncture seeks to address Qi flow abnormalities, so enhancing the body's inherent capacity to heal itself.

Exploring these fundamental principles lays the groundwork for understanding acupuncture practice, providing a look into the nuanced and comprehensive approach it takes to healing and well-being.

CHAPTER 2

Acupuncture Tools And Techniques

Instruments Used In Acupuncture

Acupuncture makes use of a variety of instruments to stimulate particular places on the body. The acupuncture needle is the principal tool. These slim, silver needles are available in a variety of lengths and gauges. To maintain safety and cleanliness, they are normally composed of stainless steel and are sterile for single use.

The Role Of Needles: Types And Sizes

The size and thickness of acupuncture needles vary. Their sizes are determined by the acupuncture sites to be addressed and the depth of insertion necessary.

Thinner needles are utilized for sensitive regions or superficial points, whilst larger needles are used for deeper points or places with more muscle tissue.

Some needles are developed for specialized treatments, such as electro acupuncture, which involves passing a moderate electric current through the needle.

Other Modalities: Cupping, Moxibustion, And Acupressure

1. Cupping: This method includes producing suction on the skin's surface by putting glass, plastic, or silicone cups. It is used to increase blood flow, relax muscular tension, and treat conditions such as pain and inflammation.

2. Moxibustion is a technique in which dried mugwort (moxa) is burnt near or on acupuncture sites. Heat is used to stimulate these spots, increasing circulation and treating certain ailments.

3. Acupressure: Acupressure, like acupuncture but without needles, involves applying pressure to particular locations

with fingers or gadgets. The goal of this therapy is to stimulate these spots to relieve pain, decrease stress, and promote general health.

Within the world of traditional Chinese medicine, each of these modalities has its own set of principles and uses. They are often used in tandem with acupuncture to offer holistic care and therapy.

Acupuncture methods and instruments are refined via intensive training and instruction. Practitioners get a thorough grasp of the body's meridian systems and acupoints, as well as how to properly utilize these modalities for a variety of health issues.

Understanding these tools and procedures is a necessary first step for individuals interested in learning about acupuncture, as it lays the groundwork for delving into the complicated and interesting therapeutic practices contained within this ancient profession.

CHAPTER 3

Acupuncture Points And Their Significance

Key Acupuncture Points And Their Functions

Acupuncture points are precise bodily sites where an acupuncturist inserts needles or uses other procedures. Each point has its medicinal powers. As an example:

• LI4 (Hegu): Located between the thumb and index finger, it is often utilized for headaches and pain relief.

• LV3 (Taichong): This foot reflexology point is related to stress reduction and emotional harmony.

- ST36 (Zusanli): Located on the lower thigh, it is used to treat digestion disorders and increase energy.

Mapping Acupuncture Points On The Body

These points are distributed along meridians, which are energy routes that run through the body. Each of the twelve major meridians corresponds to a distinct organ and is connected with certain biological activities. Understanding this map helps acupuncturists identify therapy sites.

The Five Elements And Corresponding Points

The Five Elements hypothesis (wood, fire, earth, metal, and water) is linked to acupuncture sites in traditional Chinese medicine. Each element is associated with different organs, seasons, emotions, and even colors. As an example:

• Wood (Liver/Gallbladder): Points relating to these organs may help with anger and vision problems.

• Fire (cardiac/Small Intestine): Points may be associated with happiness and influence cardiac function.

• Earth (Spleen/Stomach): Corresponding points may help with overthinking and stomach issues.

• Metal (Lung/Large Intestine): Points may be associated with grieving or respiratory health.

• Water (Kidney/Bladder): Points may help with anxiety and urinary difficulties.

CHAPTER 4

Conditions And Treatments

Common Ailments And Their Acupuncture Treatments

Acupuncture, a component of traditional Chinese medicine (TCM), provides a comprehensive approach to treating a variety of diseases. Here's a look at some common illnesses and associated acupuncture treatments:

1. Pain Control:

• Back Pain: Acupuncture may relieve chronic back pain by targeting particular spots, increasing mobility, and decreasing discomfort.

• Migraines/headaches: Treatment tries to lessen headache frequency and severity by treating underlying imbalances.

• Arthritis: Acupuncture may help treat arthritis-related joint discomfort and inflammation.

• Muscle Pain: Acupuncture relaxes muscles and promotes recovery by stimulating certain spots.

2. Mental Well-Being:

Acupuncture treatments seek to alleviate stress by modulating the body's reaction to stimuli.

• **Depression:** Acupuncture may help with depression by improving emotional equilibrium.

• **Insomnia:** By treating the underlying causes of sleep disruptions, acupuncture may help improve sleep quality.

3. Digestive Problems:

• **Acid Reflux/Indigestion:** Acupuncture may help regulate digestive function and relieve pain.

• **Irritable Bowel Syndrome (IBS):** To ease symptoms, treatment focuses on harmonizing the digestive system.

4. Female Health:

• Menstrual Problems: Acupuncture may help regulate menstrual cycles and alleviate accompanying pain.

• Menopause Symptoms: Treatment seeks to reduce hot flashes, mood swings, and sleep disruptions.

Holistic Approach: Acupuncture For Mind And Body Balance

Acupuncture considers health to be a healthy balance of mind, body, and spirit. It increases general well-being by doing the following:

1. Acupuncture strives to regulate the flow of qi (vital energy) throughout the meridian

system of the body, treating abnormalities that contribute to physical or emotional problems.

2. Acupuncture may help manage emotions by treating particular points, lowering tension and anxiety, and boosting mental clarity.

3. Acupuncture treatments regularly may assist in maintaining bodily balance, thereby averting future health problems.

4. Enhancing Vitality: Acupuncture treatments are used not just to alleviate diseases, but also to boost energy and general vitality.

Complementary Therapies: Integrating Acupuncture With Other Practices

Acupuncture is often used with other complementary treatments to improve general well-being:

1. Acupuncture combined with Chinese herbal treatments may increase the efficacy of the therapy.

2. Yoga and Tai Chi are complementary to acupuncture because they promote relaxation, flexibility, and balance.

3. Acupuncture sessions often involve food guidance to help general health and recovery.

4.   Western   Medicine   Integration: Acupuncture may enhance the effectiveness of conventional medical therapies while lowering negative effects.

Understanding typical acupuncture diseases, its holistic approach and integration with various treatments may equip newcomers with a full understanding of this ancient therapeutic therapy. It stresses the interdependence of the mind, body, and spirit in attaining holistic health and harmony.

CHAPTER 5

Preparing For An Acupuncture Session

Acupuncture treatments may be both useful and transforming. Getting ready for these sessions entails several critical steps that guarantee a safe, pleasant, and successful treatment experience.

Consultation And Assessment

An initial consultation is usually held before the acupuncture treatment. This stage is critical because it allows the acupuncturist to understand your medical history, current health issues, lifestyle, and particular concerns.

The acupuncturist may adjust the treatment plan to your specific requirements via this conversation. To acquire a thorough understanding, they may inquire about symptoms, medicines, nutrition, sleep habits, and emotional well-being.

Safety Measures And Precautions

Acupuncture safety is of the utmost importance. To avoid infections or problems, the practitioner should adhere to stringent cleanliness and sanitation practices for all equipment, especially needles. It is essential to check that the acupuncturist has the necessary credentials and follows professional norms.

They should use disposable needles and keep the area clean and sterilized.

Furthermore, it is critical to address any concerns or medical issues, such as pregnancy or bleeding disorders, with the acupuncturist ahead of time. This information aids in the modification of the treatment plan to ensure that it is safe and successful for you.

What To Expect During An Acupuncture Session

Understanding the mechanics of an acupuncture treatment might help to reduce fears. Sessions are often held in a peaceful, pleasant setting. The acupuncturist will walk you through the procedure, explaining each step and answering any questions or concerns you may have.

The procedure involves inserting tiny needles into particular acupuncture spots on your body. Because these needles are so small, their insertion usually produces very little pain, commonly characterized as a mild tingling sensation or a brief squeeze. Following needle insertion, you may feel warmth, heaviness, or a mild flow of energy in the targeted regions.

The length of the session will depend on your illness and treatment strategy. Sessions typically last 20 to 40 minutes. Following that, the practitioner may offer particular post-session care or give nutritional and lifestyle recommendations to help the therapy work more effectively.

CHAPTER 6

Acupuncture In Practice

As a therapeutic therapy, acupuncture employs sophisticated procedures that tap into the body's innate healing capacities. The use of needles, comprehension of physical feelings, and frequency of sessions constitute the foundation of this ancient medical practice.

Techniques For Proper Needle Insertion

1. Cleanliness and sterilization: Before needle insertion, it is essential to ensure appropriate cleanliness. Sterilized and single-use needles reduce the danger of infection.

2. Depth and Angle of Needle Insertion: The depth and angle of needle insertion vary depending on the targeted acupuncture point and individual anatomy. Shallow insertions may be utilized for superficial locations, whilst deeper ones can go deeper.

3. Needle Manipulation: Once the needle has been implanted, practitioners may use delicate manipulations such as spinning, elevating, or rotating the needle to elicit certain feelings or reactions.

4. Patient Comfort: Making patients comfortable is critical. Effective therapy relies on clear information about the procedure and calm.

Understanding Sensations: Responses To Acupuncture

1. Deqi Sensation: Patients may feel tingling, warmth, heaviness, or a minor discomfort as a result of the Deqi sensation. This often signifies that the needle has appropriately stimulated the acupuncture spot.

2. Different Reactions: Individuals' reactions to acupuncture might vary greatly. Some people may get rapid alleviation, while others may experience delayed results. Understanding these reactions may help determine therapy effectiveness.

3. Encourage patients to discuss their feelings during and after therapy to assist in

refining future sessions and adjust therapies to their reactions.

Duration And Frequency Of Acupuncture Sessions

1. Acupuncture treatments normally take 20 to 45 minutes, however, this might vary depending on the illness being treated and individual requirements.

2. The frequency of sessions varies depending on the condition being treated. Acute illnesses may need more frequent treatments at first, but chronic disorders may necessitate continued, but less frequent, appointments.

3. The frequency of treatment may decrease as individuals achieve relief or

improvement. However, for general well-being, periodic sessions may still be suggested.

4. Acupuncture is often used in conjunction with other therapies or treatments. Collaboration with different healthcare practitioners ensures that the patient's well-being is addressed holistically.

Acupuncture may provide extraordinary advantages when done with professionalism and a thorough grasp of the body's energy flow. Implementing appropriate approaches, analyzing physical reactions, and tailoring therapies to individual requirements all contribute to its efficacy.

CHAPTER 7

Exploring Acupuncture Schools And Traditions

Acupuncture is a discipline with many different traditions and schools of thought, each with its take on treatment and healing. Understanding these varied ways may broaden one's understanding of the depth and breadth of acupuncture.

Traditional Chinese Medicine (TCM) Practices

TCM is the basis of many acupuncture procedures. It is a holistic approach to health that focuses on the Qi (vital energy) balance inside the body. Acupuncture is part of a larger system of therapy in TCM that includes herbal medication, dietary changes, and activities like Tai Chi or Qigong. To discover imbalances and restore harmony with acupuncture, TCM diagnosis often comprises pulse-taking, tongue examination, and a complete evaluation of the patient's general health.

Variations In Acupuncture Techniques: Japanese, Korean, And Five Element Acupuncture

1. Japanese Acupuncture: Japanese acupuncture is known for its sensitive and gentle needling procedures, which often use finer needles and shallower insertions. Diagnosis and therapy, stress palpation, and sensitivity to the body's energy pathways.

2.	Korean Acupuncture: Combining components of TCM and Korean medicine, Korean acupuncture emphasizes hand acupuncture (Su Jok) and uses smaller needles to target particular spots on the hands and foot.

3.	Five-Element Acupuncture: This technique is based on ancient Chinese philosophy and focuses on the five elements—wood, fire, earth, metal, and water—as they relate to biological processes and emotions. To restore health, treatment seeks to correct imbalances in these factors.

Contemporary Approaches And Innovations

Acupuncture in the modern day has developed to include numerous treatments and adapt to the changing healthcare environment. Electro acupuncture (using electrical stimulation on needles for increased benefits), trigger point acupuncture (targeting particular knots or muscle trigger points), and scalp acupuncture (focused on sites on the scalp to treat neurological problems) are some modern methods.

Understanding these many schools and methods enables practitioners to broaden their skill set, adapt to patient demands, and investigate a variety of ideas and practices that add to the complex tapestry of acupuncture. As the subject evolves, modern practitioners often draw from different traditions to deliver thorough and successful therapies.

CHAPTER 8

Integrating Acupuncture Into Daily Life

Self-Care Practices: Acupressure And Meridian Stimulation

Acupuncture is not just used in hospitals. Learning acupressure methods is required to incorporate its ideas into everyday living. These acupuncture-derived procedures include applying pressure to certain sites on the body to help in relaxation, stress release, and minor illness relief. Exploring acupressure allows people to self-manage their health.

Understanding meridian routes and how to activate them with light massage or pressure allows practitioners to tap into their bodies' innate healing capacities. Beginners may enjoy instant advantages by demonstrating numerous easy, efficient acupressure spots for common conditions such as headaches, stress, or intestinal trouble.

Dietary Recommendations For Balancing Qi

Food is considered a kind of medication in traditional Chinese medicine. The notion of Qi balance via food choices educates newcomers about the relationship between nutrition and health. Highlighting the energetics of different meals and how they affect the body's balance instructs readers on how to preserve internal harmony.

Advising on how to include Qi-balancing foods into everyday meals encourages people to take charge of their health. Suggestions for meals that support certain organs or components may help people have a better knowledge of how the body works.

Mindfulness And Meditation In Acupuncture

Acupuncture is enhanced by mindfulness and meditation because it promotes relaxation and stress reduction. Introducing fundamental meditation techniques and how they interact with the goals of acupuncture assists beginners in obtaining mental and emotional equilibrium.

Individuals may include attentive breathing exercises and basic meditation methods suited to increase the benefits of acupuncture in their everyday routine by exploring mindful breathing exercises and simple meditation techniques. The importance of their function in soothing the mind and boosting overall wellness urges frequent participation.

Individuals may nurture holistic well-being by digging into these activities and smoothly integrating acupuncture concepts into their everyday lives.

CHAPTER 9

Ethical And Legal Aspects Of Acupuncture

Acupuncture, like any other medical treatment, is bound by ethical and legal guidelines. Here's a thorough examination of the ethical and legal implications of this ancient therapeutic practice:

Licensing And Certification Requirements

Acupuncturists must follow particular licensure and certification standards established by local regulatory organizations or governing authorities. Completing authorized educational programs, clinical training, and passing national board tests are common requirements. The chapter goes into the various licensing requirements between areas, as well as the importance of acquiring the correct certification. It highlights the significance of continuing education to retain a license, emphasizing how constant learning keeps practitioners up to speed on developing procedures and standards.

Professional Ethics And Conduct In Acupuncture Practice

Ethical principles are the foundation of acupuncture practice. This section stresses acupuncturists' ethical duties, such as confidentiality, informed consent, respect for patient autonomy, and professional limits. It discusses how to preserve professionalism, ethics, and cultural awareness while engaging with patients. The chapter covers case studies demonstrating ethical quandaries that practitioners may confront, providing ideas about ethically navigating such circumstances.

Patient Rights And Responsibilities

Understanding the rights and obligations of patients is critical for both practitioners and clients. The chapter goes over patients' rights to informed consent, privacy, and access to their medical records. It informs readers about their position in their healthcare journey, promoting active engagement, honesty in revealing information, and treatment plan adherence. It also emphasizes the significance of patient input and methods for resolving problems or complaints, establishing a patient-centered approach within the practice.

CHAPTER 10

The Future Of Acupuncture

As an ancient therapeutic practice, acupuncture has continued to grow and adapt to the changing environment of contemporary healthcare. In this chapter, we look at acupuncture's possible future, analyzing scientific advances, its function in modern healthcare, and its integration for holistic well-being.

Research And Advancements In Acupuncture

Acupuncture research is gaining traction as the desire for holistic and integrative treatment develops.

Acupuncture's physiological and neurological processes are being studied by scientists and practitioners. Researchers are mapping the brain responses to acupuncture stimulation using advanced imaging methods such as functional magnetic resonance imaging (fMRI) and electroencephalography (EEG).

Furthermore, research into the effects of acupuncture on numerous health issues is underway. Clinical studies are being done to determine its efficacy in the treatment of chronic pain and mental health issues, and even as a supplementary therapy in diseases such as cancer treatment.

Another intriguing area is the use of technology with acupuncture.

Electro acupuncture, which involves passing a tiny electric current via acupuncture needles, is being researched for its possible advantages. Wearable gadgets and smartphone apps are also on the rise to let people self-administer acupressure and monitor their overall well-being.

Acupuncture's Role In Modern Healthcare

The incorporation of acupuncture into conventional treatment is a growing trend. Acupuncture services are increasingly being offered alongside conventional therapies in many hospitals and healthcare facilities. This integration acknowledges acupuncture's potential to improve patient outcomes, notably in the treatment of pain, stress, and a variety of chronic illnesses.

Acupuncturists and Western medical practitioners are increasingly collaborating. This interdisciplinary approach promotes a more holistic and patient-centered style of treatment by allowing for a thorough knowledge of patients' health.

Acupuncture is also being recognized as valuable by health insurance companies. As more scientific evidence supports its effectiveness, some insurance plans are now covering acupuncture treatments, making it more accessible to a larger population.

Embracing Acupuncture For Holistic Well-Being

Acupuncture's future includes more than just treating specific ailments; it also includes promoting overall well-being. With a greater emphasis on preventive healthcare, acupuncture is finding a role in promoting body balance and harmony.

The stress-reduction and mood-stabilizing effects of acupuncture are acknowledged as significant components of mental health therapy. Acupuncture is being integrated into the offerings of wellness centers, spas, and integrative medicine clinics to help people on their path to holistic well-being.

Furthermore, the potential for acupuncture to improve energy, sleep quality, and digestive health aligns with the growing interest in lifestyle medicine. Acupuncture is likely to play an important role in personalized wellness plans as people seek ways to improve their health and prevent illness.

Finally, with ongoing research, increased integration into healthcare systems, and its role in promoting holistic well-being, the future of acupuncture looks promising. As we continue to decipher the mysteries of this ancient practice, its potential to contribute to a balanced and healthy lifestyle becomes clearer in the modern world.

Conclusion

Acupuncture exploration takes beginners on a fascinating journey that combines ancient wisdom with modern understanding. Acupuncture, which has its roots in various cultures' traditional healing practices, has evolved into a therapeutic science that continues to captivate individuals seeking holistic well-being.

This journey began with an introduction to the fundamentals of acupuncture, delving into its historical roots and illuminating the underlying principles that govern its effectiveness. The intricate network of meridians, the vital energy flow known as Qi, and the relationship between organ systems and these energy pathways were all crucial in understanding the essence of acupuncture.

A comprehensive understanding emerged as beginners delved into the tools and techniques used in acupuncture. The richness of acupuncture's therapeutic arsenal became clear as it progressed from the subtle art of needling, with its various types and sizes of needles, to additional modalities such as cupping, moxibustion, and acupressure.

Acupuncture points, which are the focal points of energy manipulation in the body, were thoroughly investigated. Acupuncture beginners learned about key acupuncture points, their functions, and the intricate mapping of these points throughout the body. The connection to the Five Elements improved my understanding of these points and their importance in promoting balance and harmony within the body.

The journey continued with the practical application of acupuncture, where common ailments were addressed with specific treatments. Acupuncture's holistic approach, which includes both physical and mental aspects of well-being, demonstrated its ability to provide comprehensive healing. Furthermore, acupuncture's integration with complementary therapies demonstrated its versatility in producing synergistic effects for individuals seeking a holistic and balanced lifestyle.

Beginners were introduced to ongoing research and advancements in the field as they considered the future of acupuncture. Acupuncture's growing importance in modern healthcare systems became clear, as did its ability to complement and enhance conventional medical practices. As the world recognizes the value of holistic well-being, acupuncture is poised to play an important role in shaping the future of healthcare.

Finally, for those new to acupuncture, the journey is more than just a study of ancient practices; it is a profound exploration of one's own body, mind, and spirit. As the rich tapestry of acupuncture unfolds, beginners gain not only knowledge but also a holistic approach to health and a sense of empowerment over their well-being. Acupuncture has a bright future, and as new practitioners embrace this ancient art, they contribute to its ongoing evolution and integration into the modern landscape of wellness and healing.

THE END

www.ingramcontent.com/pod-product-compliance
Lightning Source LLC
Chambersburg PA
CBHW050748260726
48661CB00001B/485